I0425908

Contents

Highlights of this Evaluation

The Health Hazard Evaluation Program received a request from the United Food and Commercial Workers union. Union officials were concerned that employees at a poultry breading plant in Georgia were experiencing asthma, bronchitis, and nasal symptoms from exposure to breading dust, which consists of flour, spices, and other ingredients.

What We Did

- We evaluated the plant in June 2009. We returned in March 2010.

- We looked at work processes, practices, and conditions.

- We took air samples for inhalable flour dust, wheat, and soy.

- We considered employees as "lower-exposure" or "higher-exposure" on the basis of their current job.

- We tested employees' blood to see if they were allergic to flour dust, wheat, garlic, onion, soybean, corn, or paprika. All of these items are used in the plant. We also tested employees for common allergens like grass and pollen.

- We surveyed employees about their job and their health. We asked them if they had symptoms of cough, asthma, or allergies.

What We Found

- The median concentration of inhalable flour dust in air was 8.21 milligrams per cubic meter in the higher-exposure group. It was 1.03 milligrams per cubic meter in the lower-exposure group.

- Most inhalable flour dust exposures were above the recommended value of 0.5 milligrams per cubic meter for flour dust. This value was set by the American Conference of Governmental Industrial Hygienists.

> We evaluated exposures to breading dust (which contains flour, spices, and other ingredients) at a poultry breading plant. Employees reported asthma, bronchitis, and nasal symptoms. We found that employees were overexposed to flour dust and other breading ingredients due to a lack of ventilation and poor work practices. Because of these high exposures some employees were sensitized to flour dust, wheat, spices, and other ingredients. We also found employees with work-related asthma symptoms, cough, and rhinoconjunctivitis symptoms. We recommend that employees wear respirators until engineering controls and work practices can reduce exposures. We also recommend that the plant start a medical surveillance program.

- Employees in the higher-exposure group were more likely than those in the lower-exposure group to report several work-related symptoms in the last 12 months. These included wheezing or whistling in the chest, problems with sneezing or a runny nose or a blocked nose without a cold, and problems with sneezing or a runny nose or a blocked nose without a cold accompanied by itchy, watery eyes.

What We Found (continued)

- Employees in the higher-exposure group were more likely than those in the lower-exposure group to be sensitized to flour dust and wheat.

- Employees who were sensitized to flour dust, wheat, corn, or onion were more likely to report work-related asthma symptoms than those who did not have these allergies.

- Work-related episodes of coughing were common among employees, regardless of sensitization.

What the Employer Can Do

- Use an enclosed system to transfer powdered ingredients to the dispensing hoppers.

- Use local exhaust ventilation to lower flour dust levels.

- Start a respiratory protection program. Respiratory protection should be used until engineering controls and work practices can reduce exposures. Exposures should be below the American Conference of Governmental Industrial Hygienists Threshold Limit Value for flour dust.

- Hire a physician to evaluate employees for respiratory symptoms before they begin work at the facility. These evaluations should be repeated periodically after that.

What Employees Can Do

- Wear the respirators provided by the company properly.

- Report any health problems that may be related to work to your supervisor or plant nurse so you can be referred for a medical evaluation.

This page left intentionally blank

Abbreviations

ACGIH®	American Conference of Governmental Industrial Hygienists
CFR	Code of Federal Regulations
HHE	Health hazard evaluation
IgE	Immunoglobulin E
IOM	Institute of Medicine
kU/L	Killiunits per liter of serum
mg/m^3	milligrams per cubic meter
NAICS	North American Industry Classification System
ND	Not detected
NIOSH	National Institute for Occupational Safety and Health
OEL	Occupational exposure limit
OSHA	Occupational Safety and Health Administration
PEL	Permissible exposure limit
REL	Recommended exposure limit
STEL	Short-term exposure limit
TLV®	Threshold limit value
TWA	Time-weighted average
WEEL™	Workplace environmental exposure level

Introduction

On April 3, 2009, the National Institute for Occupational Safety and Health (NIOSH) received a request for a health hazard evaluation (HHE) at a poultry breading plant in Georgia. The United Food and Commercial Workers union submitted the request. The request stated that employees at the plant were experiencing asthma, bronchitis, and nasal symptoms from exposure to breading dust, which consists of flour, spices, and other ingredients.

NIOSH investigators visited the plant on June 24–25, 2009. We held an opening meeting with plant managers, the corporate health and safety manager, and union representatives to discuss the HHE request. We observed work processes, practices, and workplace conditions and spoke with employees. We reviewed material safety data sheets for breading ingredients, the plant's respiratory protection program, the Occupational Safety and Health Administration (OSHA) Log of Work-Related Injuries and Illnesses Form 300 from 2005 to 2009, and environmental sampling results from 2003 to 2009. We also held confidential interviews with 47 employees to discuss health and workplace concerns. We sent an interim letter with the findings from this visit to the participants of the opening meeting. We returned to the plant on March 8–10, 2010, to further evaluate employees' exposures to breading dust.

Background

Process Description

More than 400 employees worked in production at this plant, which had two production shifts and one sanitation shift. The plant received raw chicken from deboning plants. The chicken was then breaded, flash fried, and frozen; breaded, fully cooked, and frozen; or marinated and frozen. The plant had six production lines that used interchangeable components including conveyor belts, marinating tanks, and breading and batter applicators. One line was devoted to marinating and freezing chicken.

Dry batter and breading mix supplied in paper bags of varying sizes were manually emptied into dispensing hoppers along the lines. Local exhaust ventilation on the lines could be connected to the interchangeable components as they were rearranged to accommodate the type of chicken product being produced.

Baker's Asthma

Baker's asthma is a well-known form of occupational asthma. Rhinitis (inflammation inside the nose) among bakers is common and usually precedes asthma. Conjunctivitis (inflammation of the white part of the eye and the lining of the eyelids) and skin symptoms may also occur. Atopy (the predisposition to allergy) is a risk factor for asthma, but sex, age, and smoking habits do not have a significant influence on sensitization or asthma [De Zotti et al. 1994; Baur et al. 1998; Houba et al. 1998a]. Symptoms of baker's asthma may develop months or years after first exposure, and risk increases with increasing exposure concentration. In addition to allergy, nonspecific mucous membrane and respiratory irritation also occur frequently among those exposed to flour, possibly more commonly than allergic symptoms [Houba et al. 1998b].

Wheat and other cereal flours are the main causes of baker's asthma. Wheat flour is a complex mixture that contains at least 40 antigens [Sander et al. 2001]. Epidemiologic studies have demonstrated prevalences of sensitization of 5%–28% to wheat among bakers [Houba et al. 1996]. Variability in these prevalences is due to differing methods for measuring sensitization. The prevalence of sensitization to flour dust and spices, allergy, and asthma among poultry breading workers is unknown, as is the range of exposures in this type of manufacturing environment.

Methods

Previous environmental monitoring for total dust by the plant found employee exposures that exceeded the OSHA permissible exposure limit (PEL) for particulates not otherwise regulated. Using this information and observation of plant processes, for our statistical analysis we classified employees as "lower-exposure" or "higher-exposure." The lower-exposure group included employees who worked on lines breading chicken but worked with product that was already cooked, employees on a line that did not bread chicken, and other jobs with minimal direct contact with breading dust (Table 1). The higher-exposure group included production employees who handled flour and other ingredients and uncooked breaded product (Table 1). Persons who reported prior job assignments at the plant that were in the higher-exposure group were assigned to the past higher-exposure group.

All production employees at the plant were asked to participate in our evaluation. The evaluation was designed to compare sensitization and symptoms prevalences between groups of employees with differing levels of exposure to breading dust and to characterize exposure to flour dust, wheat, and soy. Full-shift personal breathing zone air samples for inhalable flour dust, wheat, and soy were collected across job titles on all six lines. Although we did not evaluate ventilation controls, we observed use of the ventilation systems.

Employees were informed of the benefits and risks of the evaluation and gave signed consent for participation. We drew participants' blood and tested it for immunoglobulin E (IgE) antibody specific to flour dust, wheat, garlic, onion, soybean, corn, and paprika. We also tested for common aeroallergens (using the AlaTOP®) to assess atopy. A positive antibody test indicates sensitization to a specific substance.

We administered a questionnaire to all participants, asking about job title, years worked, and work department; cough; symptoms of asthma; and symptoms of rhinoconjunctivitis (nose and eye symptoms). Study participants were individually informed in writing of the results of their blood tests and what they meant.

The methods used for this evaluation are discussed in detail in Appendix A.

Table 1. Employee exposure groups*

Lower exposure	Higher exposure
Clerk in office	Bread and batter
Fork lift operator	Lay-on
Bagger operators	Oven operators
Trash dock and trash removal	Marination
Receiving employees	Foremax operators
Scale operators	Line leader
Box makers	Quality assurance technicians
Frozen shipping employees	Bone checker
Tub washers	Utility
Temperature checkers	Checker/sorter
Stackers	
Quality assurance production and support	
Packers	
Cups	
Warehouse ingredient handlers	
Graders	
Pallet jack operators	

*Employees were classified on the basis of a review of work processes, historical sampling data, and the professional judgment of NIOSH investigators.

Results

First Site Visit

Previous sampling by the plant found employee exposures to total dust (comprised mainly of flour) at concentrations that exceeded the OSHA PEL of 15 mg/m^3 for particulates not otherwise regulated. In addition to flour dust, other ingredients used in the plant have been reported in the medical literature to cause asthma including garlic, onion, soy, and corn. Spicy flour used in the plant contained paprika and capsaicin, which can cause mucous membrane and respiratory irritation.

Our review of the OSHA Logs revealed one employee diagnosed with baker's asthma in 2005. We interviewed 47 of more than 400 production employees. Twelve of the 47 were identified from a list provided by the union of 18 employees who had reported work-related symptoms; the other six on the union list were not at work at the time of our visit. The remaining 35 interviewed employees were serially selected from job categories with the greatest potential for flour dust exposure. Twenty-five reported no work-related symptoms. Of the remaining 22, six reported using an inhaler for work-related respiratory symptoms, and four reported being diagnosed with breathing problems due to flour dust. Eleven of these 22 employees reported work-related shortness of breath, 10 reported work-related cough, 9 reported work-related nasal symptoms, 8 reported work-related sneezing, 6 reported work-related eye symptoms, 5 reported work-related wheezing, and 3 reported work-related chest tightness.

Second site visit

We collected 100 personal breathing zone air samples throughout the plant. Table 2 summarizes the air sampling results for inhalable flour dust, wheat, and soy by exposure group. Tables A1–A3 in Appendix A list these personal breathing zone results by the job category observed on the day of sampling. Median airborne inhalable flour dust, wheat, and soy concentrations were higher for the higher-exposure group than the lower-exposure group, but there was overlap, and exposures were documented in all areas of the plant (Table 2). Concentrations of inhalable wheat (r = 0.89, $P < 0.01$) and soy (r = 0.79, $P < 0.01$) were positively correlated with the inhalable flour dust concentrations.

Table 2. Summary of air sampling results by exposure group as observed on the day of sampling

	Higher-exposure group	Lower-exposure group
# of PBZ samples	65	35
Inhalable flour dust		
Median	8.21 mg/m^3	1.03 mg/m^3
Range	0.59 to 93 mg/m^3	0.22 to 15 mg/m^3
Inhalable wheat		
Median	0.188 mg/m^3	0.00321 mg/m^3
Range	ND to 1.8 mg/m^3	ND to 0.44 mg/m^3
Inhalable soy		
Median	0.341 µg/m^3	ND
Range	ND to 7.2 µg/m^3	ND to 0.32 µg/m^3

Of 402 employees present during the site visit, 375 (93%) completed the questionnaire. Of these, 242 (64%) allowed their blood to be drawn.

Table 3 lists the prevalences of work-related symptoms comparing the higher-exposure group to the lower-exposure group, showing both the statistically significant (bolded) and the nonsignificant differences. Participants in the higher-exposure group were significantly more likely to report episodes of coughing, rhinitis symptoms, and rhinoconjunctivitis symptoms in the last 12 months than lower-exposure participants. Table 4 lists the prevalences of work-related symptoms comparing those currently in the higher-exposure group and those who previously held jobs in the higher-exposure group to the lower-exposure group, showing both the statistically significant (bolded) and the nonsignificant differences. Participants either currently in the higher-exposure group or who had previously held jobs in that group were significantly more likely to report asthma symptoms in the last 12 months, including wheezing or whistling in the chest and attacks of asthma, than employees in the lower-exposure group.

Of the 244 participants who reported having held other jobs at the plant, 45 reported having changed jobs for health reasons. Significantly more participants reported changing jobs for health reasons in the lower-exposure group than in the higher-exposure group (24% vs. 12%, $P = 0.01$). Twenty-three participants reported changing jobs because of respiratory tract or mucous membrane problems. Twelve of 375 participants reported having been diagnosed by a healthcare professional with allergy to flour.

Table 3. Prevalence of work-related symptoms in the last 12 months* by current exposure group

Work-related symptom	Higher-exposure group n=158–161† Number (%)	Lower-exposure group n=212–213† Number (%)	Prevalence ratio (95% confidence interval)
Episodes of coughing	43 (27)	39 (18)	**1.46 (1.00, 2.15)**‡
Asthma symptoms§	54 (34)	55 (26)	1.29 (0.94, 1.77)‡
Wheezing or whistling in chest	41 (25)	32 (15)	**1.69 (1.12, 2.58)**‡
Woken up with feeling of tightness in the chest	24 (15)	22 (10)	1.42 (0.83, 2.46)‡
Attack of asthma	11 (7)	12 (6)	1.24 (0.55, 2.76)‡
Currently taking medicine for breathing problems or asthma	22 (14)	19 (9)	1.53 (0.86, 2.77)‡
Rhinitis symptoms			
Problem with sneezing or a runny nose or a blocked nose when did not have a cold or flu	71 (44)	65 (31)	**1.45 (1.11, 1.90)**
Rhinoconjunctivitis symptoms			
Rhinitis symptoms accompanied by itchy watery eyes	51 (32)	46 (22)	**1.49 (1.06, 2.10)**

*Or since beginning current job if in that job for less than 12 months

†Denominators vary because of missing information

‡Controlled for smoking status

§Work-related asthma symptoms based upon a positive answer to one or more of four questions below it in table

Table 4. Prevalence of work-related symptoms in the last 12 months* by current and/or past exposure group

Work-related symptom	Higher-exposure group (either current or past) n=249–252† Number (%)	Lower-exposure group n=120–121† Number (%)	Prevalence ratio (95% confidence interval)
Episodes of coughing	59 (24)	22 (18)	1.25 (0.82, 1.99)‡
Asthma symptoms§	83 (33)	25 (21)	**1.61 (1.11, 2.45)‡**
Wheezing or whistling in chest	61 (24)	11 (9)	**2.65 (1.52, 5.16)‡**
Woken up with feeling of tightness in the chest	35 (14)	11 (9)	1.52 (0.83, 3.04)‡
Attack of asthma	20 (8)	2 (2)	**4.62 (1.38, 28.64)‡**
Currently taking medicine for breathing problems or asthma	32 (13)	8 (7)	1.93 (0.97, 4.39)‡
Rhinitis symptoms			
Problem with sneezing or a runny nose or a blocked nose when did not have a cold or flu	99 (39)	36 (30)	1.33 (0.97, 1.81)
Rhinoconjunctivitis symptoms			
Rhinitis symptoms accompanied by itchy watery eyes	72 (29)	24 (20)	1.46 (0.97, 2.19)

*Or since beginning current job if in that job for less than 12 months

†Denominators vary because of missing information

‡Controlled for smoking status

§Work-related asthma symptoms based upon a positive answer to one or more of four questions below it in table

Sensitization to flour dust and wheat was significantly higher among participants who reported either a current or past job in the higher-exposure group than those who never had a job in the higher-exposure group (Table 5). The prevalences of sensitization to corn, garlic, and onion were almost twice as high among participants who reported either a current or past job in the higher-exposure group than among those who never had a job in the higher-exposure group, but these were not statistically significant. Of participants in the lower-exposure group, 15% were sensitized to wheat (Table 5).

Table 5. Prevalence of sensitization to breading dust allergens by current or past exposure group

Presence of IgE specific to: Allergen	Higher-exposure group (either current or past) n=166 Number (%)	Lower-exposure group n=74 Number (%)	Prevalence ratio (95% confidence interval)
Flour dust	54 (33)	10 (14)	**2.41 (1.30, 4.46)**
Wheat	60 (36)	11 (15)	**2.43 (1.36, 4.35)**
Soybean	21 (13)	7 (9)	1.34 (0.59, 3.01)
Garlic	28 (17)	7 (9)	1.78 (0.82, 3.90)
Paprika	12 (7)	5 (7)	1.07 (0.39, 2.93)
Onion	22 (13)	5 (7)	1.96 (0.77, 4.98)
Corn	38 (23)	9 (12)	1.88 (0.96, 3.69)

The prevalences of work-related asthma symptoms were significantly higher in participants sensitized to flour dust, wheat, corn, or onion but not to soy, garlic, or paprika, than in those who were not sensitized (Tables 6, 7, 8, and 9). Participants sensitized to flour dust, wheat, or corn were significantly more likely to report having had an asthma attack in the last 12 months and to be currently taking medicine for asthma or breathing problems (Tables 6, 7, 8, and 9). Work-related episodes of coughing were common regardless of whether participants were sensitized. The prevalence of work-related allergic rhinitis and rhinoconjunctivitis symptoms did not differ significantly between those sensitized and those not sensitized to any of the tested allergens.

Table 6. Prevalence of work-related symptoms among employees sensitized and not sensitized to flour dust and wheat

Work-related symptoms	Sensitized to flour dust			Sensitized to wheat		
	No n=175–176* Number (%)	Yes n=64–66* Number (%)	P value	No n=168–169* Number (%)	Yes n=71–73* Number (%)	P value
Episodes of coughing	46 (26)	18 (27)	0.88	44 (26)	20 (27)	0.85
Asthma symptoms†	55 (31)	32 (48)	0.01	52 (31)	35 (48)	0.01
Wheezing or whistling in chest	38 (22)	26 (39)	<0.01	34 (20)	30 (41)	<0.01
Woken up with feeling of tightness in the chest	23 (13)	10 (15)	0.67	21 (12)	12 (16)	0.40
Attack of asthma	9 (5)	11 (17)	<0.01	7 (4)	13 (18)	<0.01
Currently taking medicine for breathing problems or asthma	16 (9)	19 (29)	<0.01	16 (10)	19 (26)	<0.01
Rhinitis symptoms						
Problem with sneezing or a runny nose or a blocked nose when did not have a cold or flu	78 (44)	34 (52)	0.32	73 (43)	39 (53)	0.14
Rhinoconjunctivitis symptoms						
Rhinitis symptoms accompanied by itchy watery eyes	56 (32)	25 (39)	0.29	53 (31)	28 (39)	0.23

*Denominators vary because of missing information

†Work-related asthma symptoms based upon a positive answer to one or more of four questions below it in table

Table 7. Prevalence of work-related symptoms among employees sensitized and not sensitized to corn and soy

Work-related symptoms	Sensitized to corn			Sensitized to soy		
	No n=193–194* Number (%)	Yes n=46–48* Number (%)	P value	No n=212–213* Number (%)	Yes n=27–29* Number (%)	P value
Episodes of coughing	51 (26)	13 (27)	0.93	57 (27)	7 (24)	0.75
Asthma symptoms†	62 (32)	25 (52)	0.01	74 (34)	13 (46)	0.23
Wheezing or whistling in chest	43 (22)	21 (44)	<0.01	53 (25)	11 (38)	0.14
Woken up with feeling of tightness in the chest	26 (13)	7 (15)	0.83	30 (14)	3 (10)	0.78
Attack of asthma	11 (6)	9 (19)	<0.01	18 (8)	2 (7)	1.00
Currently taking medicine for breathing problems or asthma	23 (12)	12 (25)	0.02	30 (14)	5 (18)	0.57
Rhinitis symptoms						
Problem with sneezing or a runny nose or a blocked nose when did not have a cold or flu	91 (47)	21 (44)	0.69	98 (46)	14 (48)	0.82
Rhinoconjunctivitis symptoms						
Rhinitis symptoms accompanied by itchy watery eyes	67 (35)	14 (30)	0.60	75 (35)	6 (22)	0.18

*Denominators vary because of missing information.

†Work-related asthma symptoms based upon a positive answer to one or more of four questions below it in table

Table 8. Prevalence of work-related symptoms among employees sensitized and not sensitized to garlic and onion

Work-related symptoms	Sensitized to garlic			Sensitized to onion		
	No n=205–206* Number (%)	Yes n=34–36* Number (%)	P value	No n=213–214* Number (%)	Yes n=26–28* Number (%)	P value
Episodes of coughing	52 (25)	12 (33)	0.32	55 (26)	9 (32)	0.48
Asthma symptoms†	72 (35)	15 (42)	0.45	72 (34)	15 (54)	0.04
Wheezing or whistling in chest	51 (25)	13 (36)	0.16	52 (24)	12 (43)	0.04
Woken up with feeling of tightness in the chest	28 (14)	5 (14)	1.00	29 (14)	4 (14)	1.00
Attack of asthma	16 (8)	4 (11)	0.51	15 (7)	5 (18)	0.06
Currently taking medicine for breathing problems or asthma	28 (14)	7 (19)	0.36	28 (13)	7 (25)	0.15
Rhinitis symptoms						
Problem with sneezing or a runny nose or a blocked nose when did not have a cold or flu	95 (46)	17 (47)	0.90	99 (46)	13 (46)	0.99
Rhinoconjunctivitis symptoms						
Rhinitis symptoms ccompanied by itchy watery eyes	73 (35)	8 (24)	0.17	74 (35)	7 (27)	0.44

*Denominators vary because of missing information

†Work-related asthma symptoms based upon a positive answer to one or more of four questions below it in table

Table 9. Prevalence of work-related symptoms among employees sensitized and not sensitized to paprika

Work-related symptoms	Sensitized to paprika		P value
	No n=223–224* Number (%)	Yes n=16–18* Number (%)	
Episodes of coughing	61 (27)	3 (17)	0.41
Asthma symptoms†	78 (35)	9 (50)	0.20
Wheezing or whistling in chest	57 (26)	7 (39)	0.27
Woken up with feeling of tightness in the chest	31 (14)	2 (11)	1.00
Attack of asthma‡	18 (8)	2 (11)	0.65
Currently taking medicine for breathing problems or asthma	32 (14)	3 (17)	0.73
Rhinitis symptoms			
Problem with sneezing or a runny nose or a blocked nose when did not have a cold or flu	104 (46)	8 (44)	0.87
Rhinoconjunctivitis symptoms			
Rhinitis symptoms accompanied by itchy watery eyes	77 (34)	4 (25)	0.44

*Denominators vary because of missing information.

†Work-related asthma symptoms based upon a positive answer to one or more of four questions below it in table

We found no significant difference in the prevalence of atopy between groups. Atopics were significantly more likely to be sensitized to all allergens tested (Table 10).

Table 10. Prevalence of sensitization to breading dust components, by atopy

	Atopy		P value
	Yes (n=81)	No (n=155)	
Sensitized to flour dust Number (%)	47 (58)	19 (12)	< 0.01
Sensitized to wheat Number (%)	51 (63)	21 (14)	< 0.01
Sensitized to soy Number (%)	27 (33)	2 (1)	< 0.01
Sensitized to corn Number (%)	42 (52)	4 (3)	< 0.01
Sensitized to garlic Number (%)	32 (40)	3 (2)	< 0.01
Sensitized to paprika Number (%)	17 (21)	1 (1)	< 0.01
Sensitized to onion Number (%)	26 (32)	1 (1)	< 0.01

At the time of our evaluation, employees on the hazardous materials team (mainly refrigeration and select maintenance employees) were included in the respiratory protection program. We did not review the respiratory requirements for the hazardous materials team as part of this evaluation. While production employees were not required to wear respiratory protection and were not included in the respiratory protection program, some employees used NIOSH-approved N95 filtering facepiece respirators voluntarily. We saw some employees wearing their filtering facepiece respirators incorrectly. Examples of incorrect filtering facepiece respirator use included employees wearing their respirator over a beard guard, incorrectly placing the respirator only over their mouth, and using only one strap.

The bread and batter lines were equipped with local exhaust ventilation. However, we saw instances where the local exhaust ventilation was not connected to the duct work (Figures 1, 2, 3, and 4). Local exhaust ventilation was absent from the dispensing hoppers at the point where dry ingredients were transferred from paper bags to the dispensing hoppers (Figure 5). We observed that many of the local exhaust ventilation collection points between the breading line machines did not collect all the flour dust, evidenced by dust accumulation in the immediate work area (Figure 4). We observed product conveyers that were neither enclosed nor equipped with local exhaust ventilation (Figures 3, 4, and 6). On batter and bread hoppers and breading machines that were enclosed, access doors were not closed (Figure 5 and 7), resulting in dust escaping because of machine vibration.

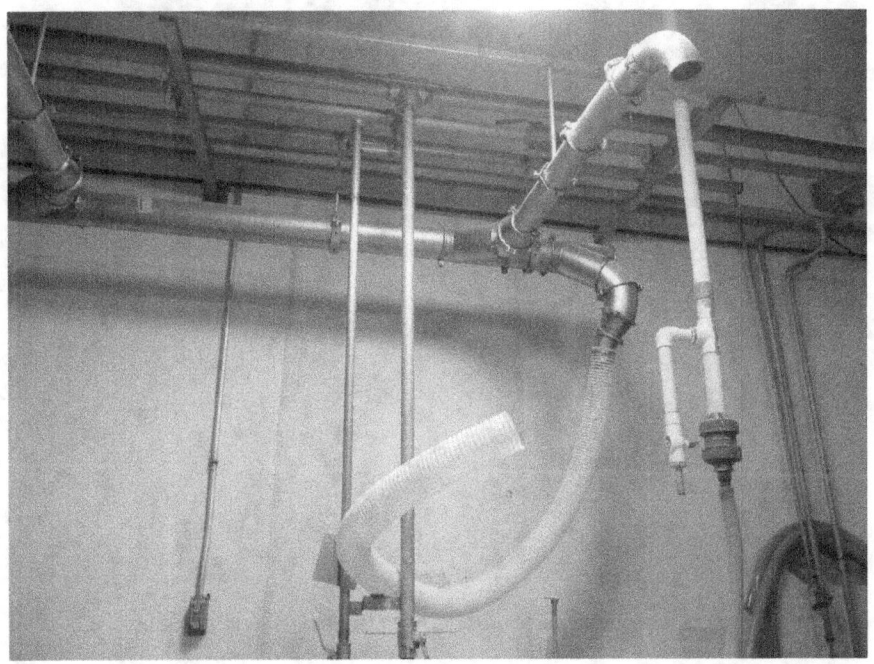

Figure 1. Disconnected and uncapped local exhaust ventilation duct on line one.

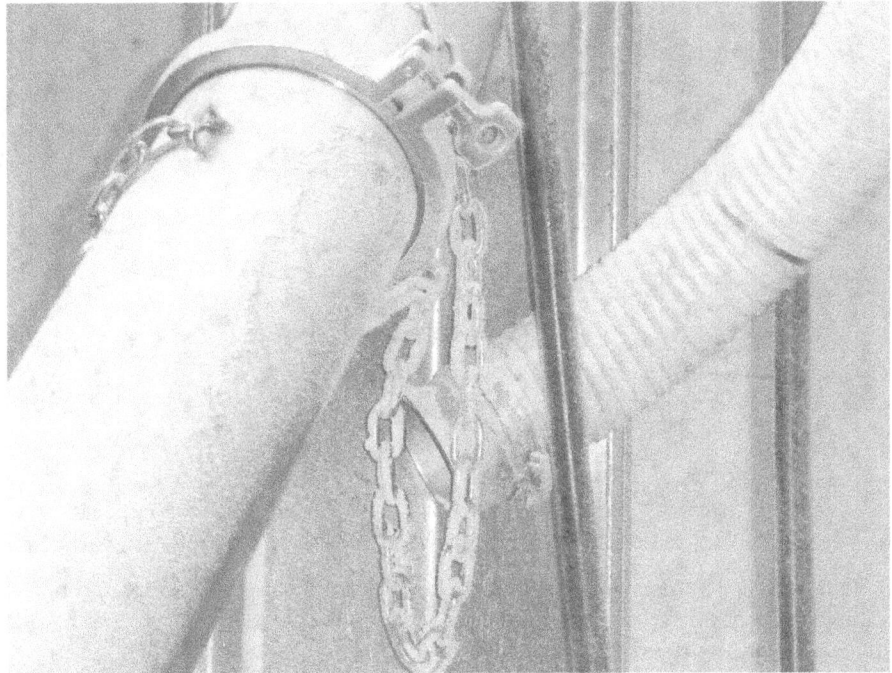

Figure 2. Disconnected and uncapped local exhaust ventilation duct on line one.

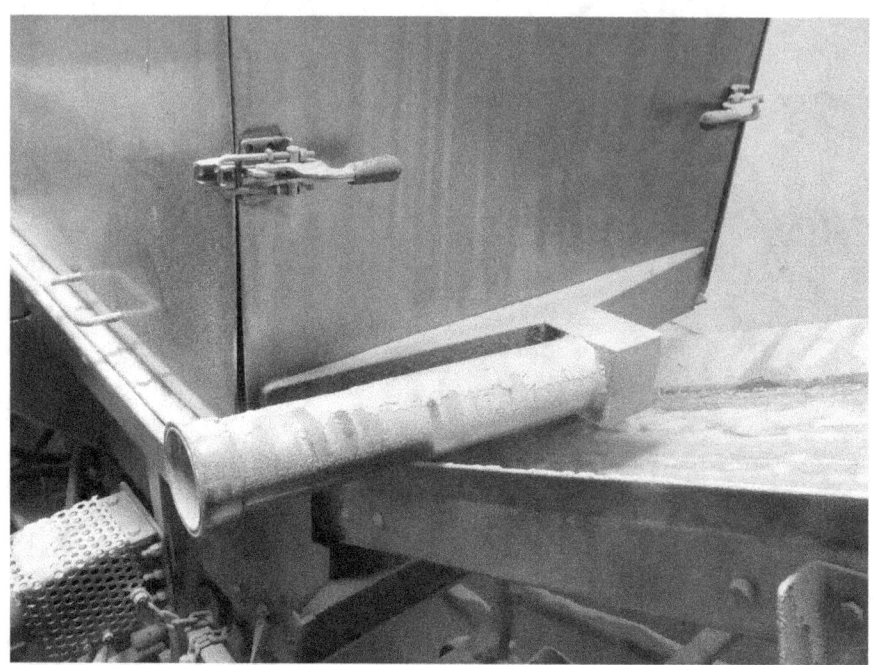

Figure 3. Local exhaust ventilation attachment not in use on breader.

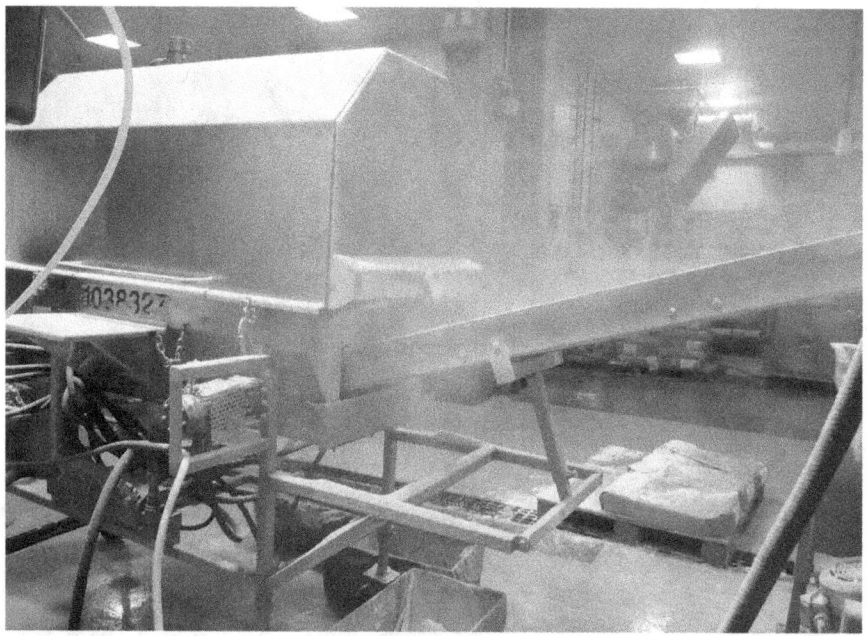

Figure 4. Local exhaust ventilation attachment not in use on breader and non-enclosed product conveyer belt.

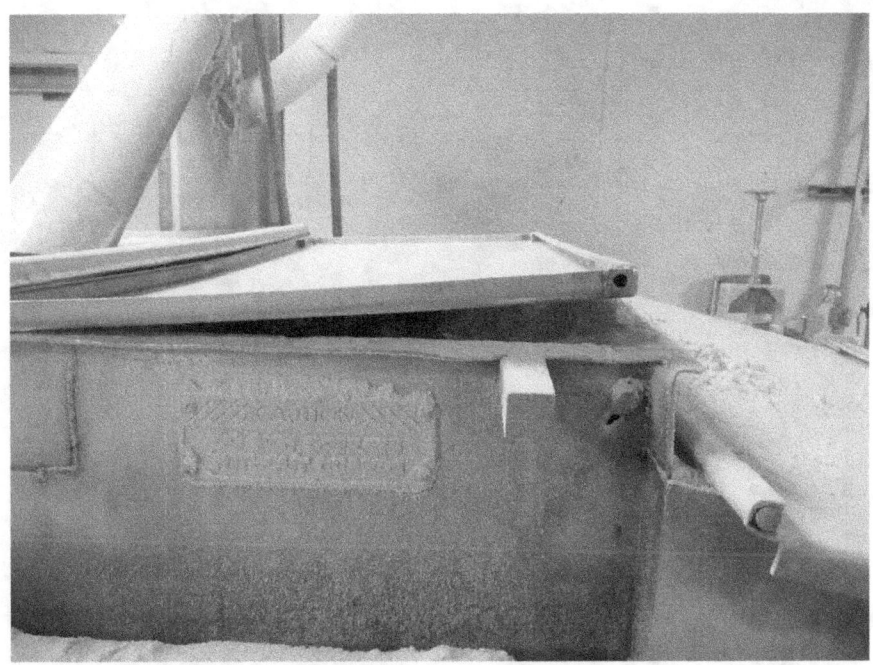

Figure 5. Dispensing hopper lid on breading machine.

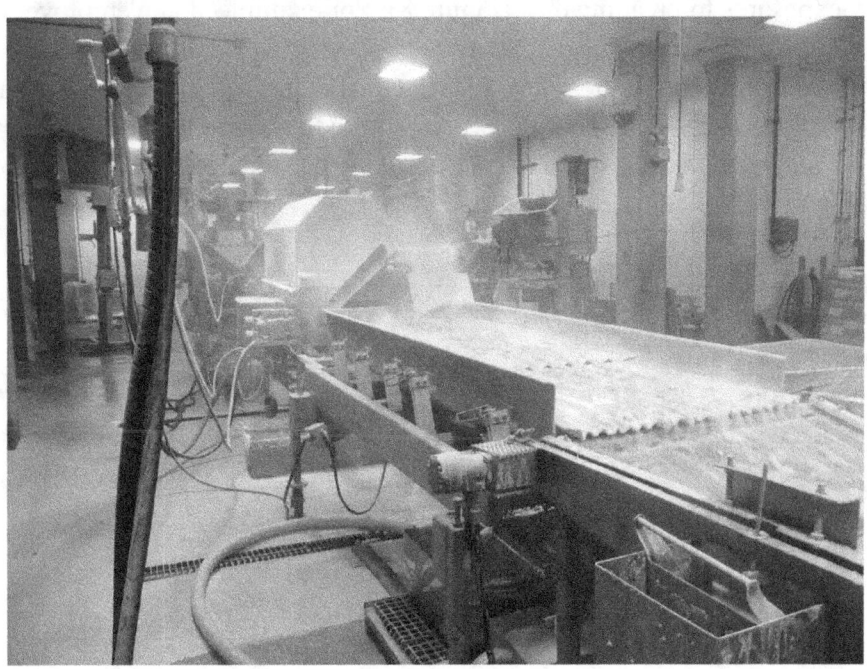

Figure 6. Unenclosed conveyor belt without local exhaust ventilation and transfer point between machines.

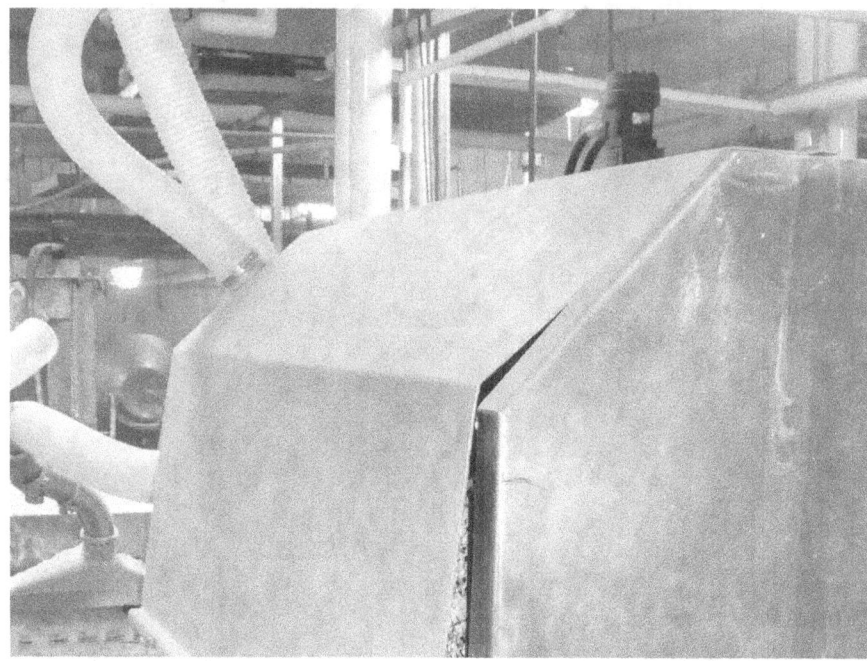

Figure 7. Open enclosure on breading machine.

We observed employees using poor techniques to transfer dry powdered ingredients, resulting in unnecessary exposures to breading dust (Figure 8). For example, some employees transferred dry ingredients to overhead hoppers or hoppers in difficult to reach locations. This often required them to place their head into the dust cloud generated by the transfer. We also observed employees transferring dry powdered ingredients into the hoppers using quick movements that generated visible dust clouds. These practices increased exposure to the airborne breading dust.

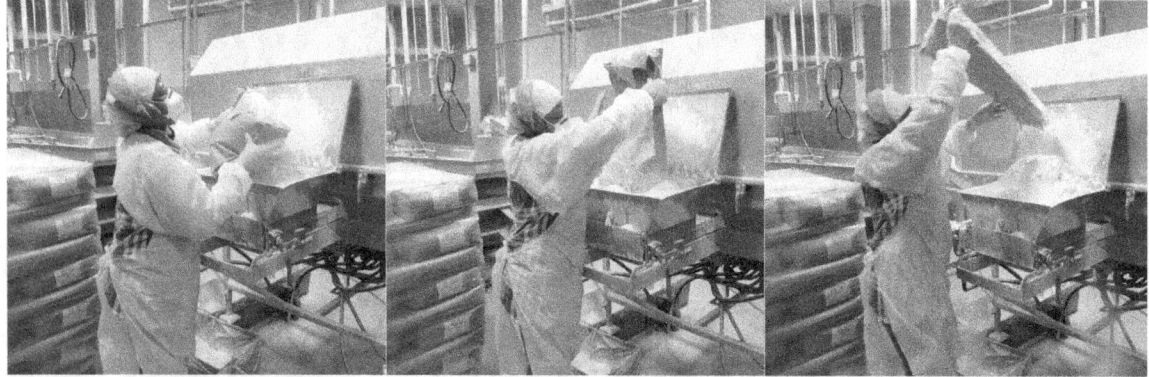

Figure 8. Employee transferring dry powdered ingredients into a breading machine hopper at breathing zone height.

Discussion

A health hazard existed at this plant from exposure to breading dust. Personal breathing zone air sampling showed that employees in almost all areas of the plant had the potential for exposure to flour dust levels above the American Conference of Governmental Industrial Hygienists (ACGIH®) threshold limit value (TLV®) for flour dust. We compared our sampling results to the ACGIH TLV because it is specific to flour dust and was established to minimize the potential for wheat flour sensitization. At the time of this evaluation the company evaluated employee exposures by comparing them to the less protective OSHA PEL for particulates not otherwise regulated. We believe this practice led to the high prevalences of sensitization to flour dust, wheat, spices, and other ingredients; and to work-related asthma symptoms, cough, and rhinoconjunctivitis. Exposures to flour dust in the plant must be reduced to prevent adverse health effects and minimize worsening of existing symptoms and disease.

The prevalence of sensitization to wheat among the higher-exposure group in this evaluation (36%) is higher than that found in studies of bakers (5%–28%) [Houba et al. 1996; Baatjies et al. 2010]. The prevalence of sensitization to wheat among participants in the lower-exposure group (15%) was within the range found in bakers and higher than in the general population (1.2% to 4.1%) [Houba et al. 1996; Gautrin et al. 1997; Biagini et al. 2004]. This is consistent with our data showing exposure to flour dust and wheat throughout the plant.

We placed participants into exposure groups on the basis of our observations of their work, a review of historical exposure data collected by the plant, and our professional judgment, but we may have misclassified some employees. Additionally, after reviewing our personal breathing zone results, we concluded that few, if any, plant employees are unexposed to flour dust and other breading ingredients.

As a result of our classification strategy, although the higher-exposure group had a median inhalable flour dust concentration several times higher than the lower-exposure group the exposures were overlapping. Moreover, airborne concentrations of inhalable flour dust and wheat for the higher-exposure group in our evaluation were much higher and those of our lower-exposure group were similar or higher than those found in Belgian bakeries [Bulat et al. 2004]. Median inhalable flour dust concentrations in a study of 55 bakeries in the United Kingdom were midway between those of our two exposure groups; however, peak exposures were much higher in our higher-exposure group [Elms et al. 2005]. Inhalable flour dust and wheat concentrations were also much higher than personal breathing zone samples from supermarket bread bakers in South Africa, even for the lower-exposure group [Baatjies et al. 2010]. Exposures to flour dust occurred throughout the plant, including areas where batter or breading mixes were not used. While the inhalable flour dust sampling method is a weight gain analysis not specific to flour dust, the presence of wheat allergens on the samples confirmed that flour dust was present in those areas.

While 23 participants reported changing jobs because of respiratory tract or mucous membrane problems related to flour dust and 12 participants reported having been diagnosed with allergy to flour by a healthcare professional, the burden of suspected disease related to exposure to flour dust and other ingredients is much higher. Thirty-four percent of higher-exposure and 26% of lower-exposure group participants had work-related asthma symptoms, yet only 14% of the higher-exposure group and 9% of the lower-exposure group were taking asthma medicine. This suggests undiagnosed occupational asthma among employees. In addition, 37% of participants reported symptoms of occupational allergic rhinitis. Participants with atopy were significantly more likely to be sensitized to wheat and other ingredients, consistent with past studies of bakery and food allergy.

Work-related asthma symptoms were significantly more common in participants sensitized to flour dust, wheat, corn, or onion than in those who were not sensitized. In addition to baker's asthma, IgE-mediated asthma and other allergic disease due to corn, soybean, onion, garlic, and paprika have been reported in the medical literature [Park and Nahm 1997; Schöll and Jensen-Jarolim 2004; Cummings et al. 2010]. Sensitization to these allergens was common among participants, regardless of exposure group.

Work-related episodes of coughing were common among participants, regardless of sensitization, likely representing general irritation from dust. Prevalences of work-related allergic rhinitis and rhinoconjunctivitis symptoms were also reported by more than 20% of all participants, regardless of sensitization. Work-related irritation symptoms are reported in the medical literature to be more common than allergic symptoms among employees exposed to flour dust.

Inhalable wheat ($r = 0.89$) and inhalable soy ($r = 0.79$) were positively correlated with the inhalable flour dust concentrations. Other studies have also documented significant correlation between inhalable wheat and inhalable flour dust [Baatjies et al. 2010; Page et al. 2010]. This supports the use of inhalable flour dust sampling for monitoring exposures instead of the more complicated and expensive inhalable wheat sampling.

The preferred method to control flour dust exposures is through engineering controls. The plant management implemented local exhaust ventilation, but it was inadequate and exposures still remain high. We did not quantitatively evaluate the local exhaust ventilation as part of this HHE, but we did note that some local exhaust ventilation units were not connected and were not adequately controlling exposures. Until engineering controls are documented to lower exposures below the ACGIH TLV, respiratory protection should be worn throughout the plant.

The implementation of a respiratory protection program and the selection of respirators should follow the OSHA respiratory protection standard [29 CFR 1910.134] and the NIOSH respirator selection logic [NIOSH 2004]. Once engineering controls (i.e., ventilation changes) have been implemented, employees' exposures should be reevaluated. Once exposures have been reduced, the respiratory protection requirement should be reassessed using the NIOSH respirator selection logic because some jobs may no longer need respiratory protection and others may need lower levels of protection. For jobs that still require respiratory protection, task-based exposures should be evaluated to identify specific tasks that require respirators and those that may not. This may also help to prioritize engineering control recommendations.

Conclusions

Nearly all plant employees whom we sampled were overexposed to flour dust from the batter mixes and breading dusts. Dust concentrations for all employees we sampled, except frozen shipping and some receiving and line 6 employees, exceeded the ACGIH TLV for flour dust during our evaluation. Lack of or inadequate ventilation controls and poor work practices contributed to high flour dust exposures. Sensitization to flour dust, wheat, spices, and other ingredients was highly prevalent. There were high prevalences of work-related asthma symptoms, cough, and rhinoconjunctivitis among all employees. Our evaluation suggests that some employees have undiagnosed occupational asthma.

Recommendations

On the basis of our findings, we recommend the actions listed below. We encourage the poultry breading plant to use a labor-management health and safety committee or working group to discuss our recommendations and develop an action plan. Those involved in the work can best set priorities and assess the feasibility of our recommendations for the specific situation at this poultry breading plant.

Our recommendations are based on an approach known as the hierarchy of controls (Appendix C: Occupational Exposure Limits and Health Effects). This approach groups actions by their likely effectiveness in reducing or removing hazards. In most cases, the preferred approach is to eliminate hazardous materials or processes and install engineering controls to reduce exposure or shield employees. Until such controls are in place, or if they are not effective or feasible, administrative measures and personal protective equipment may be needed.

Engineering Controls

Engineering controls reduce exposures to employees by removing the hazard from the process or placing a barrier between the hazard and the employee. Engineering controls are very effective at protecting employees without placing primary responsibility of implementation on the employee.

1. Evaluate the local exhaust ventilation systems to determine if they can be altered to lower dust exposures below the ACGIH TLV for flour dust. If the current systems cannot achieve these specified limits, modify or replace the systems.

2. Use a pneumatic transfer system equipped with a bag dump station to transfer powdered ingredients to the dispensing hoppers. The system should be equipped

with a negative pressure bag dump station that locally captures and exhausts airborne dust. This will eliminate the need for employees to add powdered ingredients to the dispensing hoppers using awkward postures and reduce unnecessary dust exposure.

Administrative Control

The term administrative controls refers to employer-dictated work practices and policies to reduce or prevent hazardous exposures. Their effectiveness depends on employer commitment and employee acceptance. Regular monitoring and reinforcement are necessary to ensure that policies and procedures are followed consistently.

1. Institute a medical surveillance program for employees who are exposed to batter and breading mixes. At a minimum, use a medical questionnaire that focuses on skin, mucous membrane, and respiratory symptoms that are work related. The questionnaire should be given prior to placement in a job with batter and breading mix exposure and periodically thereafter. The medical surveillance program should be supervised by a physician experienced in occupational medicine or allergy.

2. Employees should report work-related skin, eye, and respiratory symptoms to their supervisor. Employees who report work-related symptoms should be evaluated by a physician experienced in occupational medicine or allergy. If employees develop occupational rhinitis or asthma, they should be removed from exposure to flour dust and placed in a job without flour dust exposure while maintaining their earnings, seniority, and other rights and benefits.

3. Encourage employees to use slow, smooth movements when handling powdered ingredients to keep dust concentrations low. Transport distances between the paper bag and dispensing hoppers should be kept to a minimum. The height at which powdered ingredients are dropped into a container should also be kept to a minimum. Opening both ends of paper bags will reduce the amount of dust that becomes airborne when emptied.

Personal Protective Equipment

Personal protective equipment is the least effective means for controlling hazardous exposures. Proper use of personal protective equipment requires a comprehensive program and requires a high level of employee involvement and commitment. The right personal protective equipment must be chosen for each hazard. Supporting programs such as training, change-out schedules, and medical assessment may be needed. Personal protective equipment should not be the sole method for controlling hazardous exposures. Rather, personal protective equipment should be used until effective engineering and administrative controls are in place.

1. Use respiratory protection until engineering controls and work practices can be implemented that reduce employee exposure below the ACGHI TLV for flour dust. Implementation should follow the OSHA respiratory protection standard [29 CFR 1910.134]. Respiratory protection should be used as a temporary control, not a permanent solution to controlling dust exposures.

On the basis of our air sampling data, bread and batter operators should wear particulate respirators with a minimum assigned protection factor of 1,000. Using the NIOSH respirator selection logic this would mean using a pressure-demand supply-air respirator equipped with a half-mask [NIOSH 2004]. According to OSHA, a full facepiece powered air purifying respirator also provides an assigned protection factor of 1,000 [OSHA 2009]. Line leaders, lay-on employees, and oven operators should wear particulate respirators with a minimum assigned protection factor of 50. All other employees in the production areas of the plant should wear respirators with a minimum assigned protection factor of 10. Because these two assigned protection categories include several types of respirators we suggest reviewing the NIOSH respirator selection logic http://www.cdc.gov/niosh/docs/2005-100/pdfs/2005-100.pdf and the OSHA Assigned Protection Factors for the Revised Respiratory Protection Standard http://www.osha.gov/Publications/3352-APF-respirators.pdf [NIOSH 2004; OSHA 2009].

Appendix A: Tables

Table A1. Personal breathing zone air sampling results for inhalable flour dust

Exposure group	Position description	# samples	Concentration (mg/m³)		
			Median	Min	Max
Lower	Bagger operator or twin bagger operator	3	1.03	0.66	1.0
	Frozen shipping	3	0.265	0.22*	0.31
	Grader	2	2.00	1.1	2.9
	Ingredients warehouse	1	1.11	—	—
	Packer	6	1.42	0.75	15
	Pallet jack or manual pallet jack operator	2	1.25	1.2	1.3
	Quality assurance production and support	4	1.01	0.80	1.3
	Receiving	2	0.376	0.24*	0.51
	Stack off or stacker	1	0.785	—	—
	Temperature checker	1	0.800	—	—
	Line 6	7	0.655	0.49	2.7
	Cups	3	1.09	0.64	1.1
Higher	Bone checker marination	3	2.23	1.4	2.6
	Bread and batter operator	14	32.2	11	93
	Foremax operator	2	5.63	5.3	6.0
	Lay-on	23	9.72	1.5	28
	Marination	2	2.62	1.7	3.6
	Oven operator	6	3.92	1.2	22
	Quality assurance technicians	6	1.10	0.59	8.3
	Lay-on post fryer	7	3.16	1.7	39
	Line leader	2	10.4	8.2	13

Min = minimum
Max = maximum
*Trace: between the minimum detectible concentration and minimum quantifiable concentration

Table A2. Personal breathing zone air sampling results for inhalable wheat

Exposure group	Position description	# samples	Concentration (mg/m³)		
			Median	Min	Max
Lower	Bagger operator or twin bagger operator	3	0.00463	*	0.0053
	Frozen shipping	3	0.00321	*	0.013
	Grader	2	0.0225	0.00047	0.044
	Ingredients warehouse	1	0.0000254	—	—
	Packer	6	0.00788	*	0.44
	Pallet jack or manual pallet jack operator	2	0.0391	0.013	0.065
	Quality assurance production and support	4	0.0120	0.00049	0.045
	Receiving	2	*	*	*
	Stack off or stacker	1	0.0176	—	—
	Temperature checker	1	0.00622	—	—
	Line 6	7	*	*	0.027
	Cups	3	*	*	0.016
Higher	Bone checker marination	3	0.0470	0.029	0.054
	Bread and batter operator	14	0.614	0.30	1.8
	Foremax operator	2	0.343	0.21	0.48
	Lay-on	23	0.188	*	0.66
	Marination	2	0.0273	0.019	0.035
	Oven operator	6	0.147	0.0034	0.32
	Quality assurance technicians	6	0.0185	*	0.25
	Lay-on post fryer	7	0.0589	0.012	0.96
	Line leader	2	0.197	0.14	0.25

Min = minimum
Max = maximum
*Not detected

Table A3. Personal breathing zone air sampling results for inhalable soy

Exposure group	Position description	# samples	Concentration (µg/m³)		
			Median	Min	Max
Lower	Bagger operator or twin bagger operator	3	*	*	*
	Frozen shipping	3	*	*	0.022
	Grader	2	*	*	*
	Ingredients warehouse	1	*	—	—
	Packer	6	*	*	0.32
	Pallet jack or manual pallet jack operator	2	*	*	*
	Quality assurance production and support	4	*	*	*
	Receiving	2	0.0168	*	0.034
	Stack off or stacker	1	*	—	—
	Temperature checker	1	*	—	—
	Line 6	7	0.0120	*	0.041
	Cups	3	*	*	*
Higher	Bone checker marination	3	*	*	*
	Bread and batter operator	14	1.55	*	7.2
	Foremax operator	2	0.133	0.12	0.14
	Lay-on	23	0.414	*	1.2
	Marination	2	0.121	*	0.24
	Oven operator	6	0.146	*	0.43
	Quality assurance technicians	6	0.00499	*	0.80
	Lay-on post fryer	7	0.0823	*	2.3
	Line leader	2	0.178	*	0.36

Min = minimum
Max = maximum
*Not detected

Appendix B: Methods

Study Population

We asked all employees to participate in order to compare sensitization and symptom prevalences between groups of employees with differing levels of exposure to flour dust and spices. We also wanted to characterize exposure in different departments.

Informed Consent and Notification

All potential study participants were given a consent form to read and sign. Each study participant was informed in writing of his or her own blood test results and what they meant.

Biological Samples

Approximately 15 milliliters of whole blood was collected from each participant. Venipuncture was performed by a physician or a trained technician following the universal precautions for working with blood and blood products specified by the Centers for Disease Control and Prevention [CDC 1998] and OSHA [29 CFR 1910.1030]. After venipuncture, the blood was centrifuged and the serum transported to the NIOSH laboratory for analysis.

Specific IgE to flour dust, wheat, soybean, corn, paprika, garlic, and onion allergens was measured using an IMMULITE® 2000 3gAllergy™ instrument (DPC, Los Angeles, California). The IMMULITE 2000 is a Food and Drug Administration-cleared enzyme-enhanced chemiluminescent enzyme immunoassay that quantifies specific IgE antibody. The IMMULITE 2000 has a cutoff of 0.10 killiunits per liter of serum (kU/L) IgE. The insert for the Immulite 3gAllergy™ Specific IgE Universal Kit describes two scoring systems, both of which classify specific IgE levels > 0.10 kU/L–0.34 kU/L (standard classification) and > 0.11 kU/L–0.24 kU/L (extended classification) as very low.

The IMMULITE 2000 AlaTOP Allergy Screen (12 allergens) is a Food and Drug Administration-cleared qualitative chemiluminescent enzyme-labeled sequential immunoassay. The 12 allergens included on the matrix are *Dermatophagoides pteronyssinus* (dust mite), cat epithelium, dog dander, *Cynodon dactylon* (Bermuda grass), *Phleum pretense* (timothy grass), *Penicillium notatum*, *Alternaria tenuis*, *Ambrosia artemisiifolia* (common ragweed), *Plantago lanceolata* (English plantain), *Parietaria officinalis* (wall pellitory), *Betula papyrifera* (paper birch), and *Cryptomeria japonica* (Japanese cedar). A reactive result indicates that antibodies to one or more of the component allergens in the panel are present and the tested individual is classified as atopic. A nonreactive result indicates nondetectable antibodies to the component allergens.

Questionnaire

We administered a questionnaire to all study participants that included questions about their workplace, job duties, medical history, and current respiratory and eye symptoms. Questions concerning work-related rhinoconjunctivitis (allergic eye and nose symptoms) are derived from International Study of Asthma and Allergies in Childhood [Asher et al. 1995]. The respiratory questions, including validated questions on asthma symptoms from the European Community Respiratory Health Survey [Grassi et al. 2003], included the following:

1. Have you been woken up with a feeling of tightness in your chest at any time in the last 12 months?

2. Have you had an attack of asthma in the last 12 months?

3. Are you currently taking any medicine (including inhalers or pumps, aerosols, or tablets) for breathing problems or asthma?

4. Have you had wheezing or whistling in your chest at any time in the last 12 months?

A positive response on any of these questions has a sensitivity of 75% and a specificity of 80% for asthma symptoms on the basis of a clinical examination with IgE testing against common allergens, spirometry, and methacholine challenge testing. We modified these questions by adding "or since beginning your current position if in that position less than 12 months," because some participants had not been in their current position for 12 months. If a participant responded positively to any of these questions, they were classified as having asthma symptoms. In addition, we added questions about changes in symptoms or medication use on days off work or on vacation. If the participant responded that symptoms improved on days off work or on vacation, or that medication use or asthma attacks were less frequent on days off or on vacation, then their symptoms were classified as work related.

Exposure Assessment

Personal breathing zone air sampling was used to characterize employees' exposure to flour dust, wheat, and soy. Full-shift personal breathing zone air samples for inhalable flour dust were collected across job titles on all six lines using IOM samplers with Teflon® filters (pore size 1.0 micron with laminated polytetrafluoroethylene support). IOM samplers were connected to personal sampling pumps calibrated to a flow rate of 2 liters per minute. Filter samples were changed throughout the shift to prevent overloading.

The inhalable flour dust samples were stored at ambient temperatures in sealed containers to prevent additional exposure to moisture during storage and shipment. The samples were first analyzed by the NIOSH contract lab for inhalable flour dust (weight gain). The inhalable flour dust samples had a limit of detection of 100 micrograms and a limit of quantitation of 360 micrograms. Following the weight gain analysis, the inhalable flour dust samples were then shipped to the Institute for Risk Assessment Sciences, University of Utrecht, Utrecht, Netherlands, where they were analyzed using the methods outlined below for inhalable wheat and soy allergens.

Wheat and soy allergens were recovered from the filters by extraction with phosphate-buffered saline. Concentrations of wheat were measured in the extract by inhibition immunoassay, using a pool of human immunoglobulin G4 and rabbit immunoglobulin G polyclonal antibodies [Bogdanovic et al. 2006]. The soy allergens were measured using a sandwich enzyme immunoassay with rabbit immunoglobulin G antibodies [Gomez-Olles et al. 2007]. The wheat samples had a limit of detection of 15% inhibition, and the soy was 0.1 optical density above the blank on the plate.

Statistical Analysis

SAS Version 9.1.3 software (SAS Institute, Cary, North Carolina) was used for the statistical analyses. Results with P values ≤ 0.05 were considered statistically significant. Medians were reported for personal breathing zone air samples because some distributions were skewed, and others were not. Prevalence ratios were used to compare prevalences between exposure groups. A prevalence ratio greater than 1 indicates a positive relationship between a having a symptom/sensitization and being in the higher-exposure group. Along with the prevalence ratio, a 95% confidence interval for the prevalence ratio was calculated. The prevalence ratio is considered statistically significant if the 95% confidence interval does not include the number 1. Chi square or Fisher's exact tests were used to compare the prevalence of sensitization to allergens between participants with and those without atopy and to compare symptom prevalences for those with and without sensitization to specific allergens. Spearman's correlation coefficient was used to determine the correlation between inhalable dust concentrations and soy and wheat concentrations.

Personal breathing zone air samples were corrected by subtracting the median value of the field blanks. When the field blank correction resulted in a negative value a value of zero was used in the statistical analysis, and the results were reported as not detected. Because of the lack of a reported limit of detection, inhalable wheat and soy samples were analyzed statistically using a zero when the results were reported as not detected.

Appendix C: Occupational Exposure Limits and Health Effects

NIOSH investigators refer to mandatory (legally enforceable) and recommended occupational exposure limits (OELs) for chemical, physical, and biological agents when evaluating workplace hazards. OELs have been developed by federal agencies and safety and health organizations to prevent adverse health effects from workplace exposures. Generally, OELs suggest levels of exposure that most employees may be exposed to for up to 10 hours per day, 40 hours per week, for a working lifetime, without experiencing adverse health effects. However, not all employees will be protected if their exposures are maintained below these levels. Some may have adverse health effects because of individual susceptibility, a preexisting medical condition, or a hypersensitivity (allergy). In addition, some hazardous substances act in combination with other exposures, with the general environment, or with medications or personal habits of the employee to produce adverse health effects. Most OELs address airborne exposures. But, some substances can be absorbed directly through the skin and mucous membranes.

Most OELs are expressed as a time-weighted average (TWA) exposure. A TWA refers to the average exposure during a normal 8- to 10-hour workday. Some chemical substances and physical agents have recommended short-term exposure limits (STEL) or ceiling values. Unless otherwise noted, the STEL is a 15-minute TWA exposure. It should not be exceeded at any time during a workday. The ceiling limit should not be exceeded at any time.

In the United States, OELs have been established by federal agencies, professional organizations, state and local governments, and other entities. Some OELs are legally enforceable limits; others are recommendations.

- The U.S. Department of Labor OSHA PELs (29 CFR 1910 [general industry]; 29 CFR 1926 [construction industry]; and 29 CFR 1917 [maritime industry]) are legal limits. These limits are enforceable in workplaces covered under the Occupational Safety and Health Act of 1970.

- NIOSH RELs are recommendations based on a critical review of the scientific and technical information and the adequacy of methods to identify and control the hazard. NIOSH RELs are published in the NIOSH Pocket Guide to Chemical Hazards [NIOSH 2010]. NIOSH also recommends risk management practices (e.g., engineering controls, safe work practices, employee education/training, personal protective equipment, and exposure and medical monitoring) to minimize the risk of exposure and adverse health effects.

- Other OELs commonly used and cited in the United States include (a) the TLVs, which are recommended by ACGIH, a professional organization, and (b) the Workplace environmental exposure levels (WEELs), which are recommended by the American Industrial Hygiene Association, another professional organization. The TLVs and WEELs are developed by committee members of these associations from a review of the published, peer-reviewed literature. These OELs are not consensus standards. TLVs are considered voluntary exposure guidelines for use by industrial hygienists and others trained in this discipline "to assist in the control of health hazards" [ACGIH 2012]. WEELs have been established for some chemicals "when no other legal or authoritative limits exist" [AIHA 2011].

Outside the United States, OELs have been established by various agencies and organizations and include legal and recommended limits. The Institut für Arbeitsschutz der Deutschen Gesetzlichen Unfallversicherung (IFA, Institute for Occupational Safety and Health of the German Social Accident Insurance) maintains a database of international OELs from European Union member states, Canada (Québec), Japan, Switzerland, and the United States. The database, available at http://www.dguv.de/ifa/en/gestis/limit_values/index.jsp, contains international limits for more than 1,500 hazardous substances and is updated periodically.

OSHA requires an employer to furnish employees a place of employment free from recognized hazards that cause or are likely to cause death or serious physical harm [Occupational Safety and Health Act of 1970 (Public Law 91–596, sec. 5(a)(1))]. This is true in the absence of a specific OEL. It also is important to keep in mind that OELs may not reflect current health-based information.

When multiple OELs exist for a substance or agent, NIOSH investigators generally encourage employers to use the lowest OEL when making risk assessment and risk management decisions. NIOSH investigators also encourage use of the hierarchy of controls approach to eliminate or minimize workplace hazards. This includes, in order of preference, the use of (1) substitution or elimination of the hazardous agent, (2) engineering controls (e.g., local exhaust ventilation, process enclosure, dilution ventilation), (3) administrative controls (e.g., limiting time of exposure, employee training, work practice changes, medical surveillance), and (4) personal protective equipment (e.g., respiratory protection, gloves, eye protection, hearing protection). Control banding, a qualitative risk assessment and risk management tool, is a complementary approach to protecting employee health. Control banding focuses on how broad categories of risk should be managed. Information on control banding is available at http://www.cdc.gov/niosh/topics/ctrlbanding/. This approach can be applied in situations where OELs have not been established or can be used to supplement existing OELs. Below we provide the OELs and surface contamination limits for the compounds we measured, as well as a discussion of the potential health effects from exposure to these compounds.

Flour Dust

Neither NIOSH nor OSHA has a specific occupational exposure limit for flour dust. OSHA does have a PEL for particulates not otherwise regulated of 15 milligrams per cubic meter for total dust, and 5 milligrams per cubic meter for respirable dust. However, our opinion is that the OSHA PEL for particulates not otherwise regulated is inappropriate for flour because that PEL is intended for biologically "inert" dusts. For evaluating exposure, we recommend the ACGIH TLV, or another occupational exposure limit specific to flour dust, because flour dust is an allergen and not an inert dust. The ACGIH TLV for inhalable flour dust is 0.5 milligrams per cubic meter, expressed as a TWA for up to an 8-hour workday. British Columbia, Ontario, Hong Kong, and Ireland have the same occupational exposure limit for flour dust. No occupational exposure limits specific for wheat or spices have been developed.

References

ACGIH [2012]. 2012 TLVs® and BEIs®: threshold limit values for chemical substances and physical agents and biological exposure indices. Cincinnati, OH: American Conference of Governmental Industrial Hygienists.

AIHA [2011]. AIHA 2011 Emergency response planning guidelines (ERPG) & workplace environmental exposure levels (WEEL) handbook. Fairfax, VA: American Industrial Hygiene Association.

Asher MI, Anderson HR, Beasley R, Crane J, Martinez F, Mitchell EA, Peace N, Sibbald B, Stewart AW, Strachan D, Weiland SK, Williams HC [1995]. International study of asthma and allergies in childhood (ISAAC): rationale and methods. Eur Resp J 8(3):483–491.

Baatjies R, Meijster T, Lopata A, Sander I, Raulf-Heimsoth M, Heederik D, Jeebhay M [2010]. Exposure to flour dust in South African supermarket bakeries: modeling of baseline measurements of an intervention study. Ann Occup Hyg 54(3):309–318.

Baur X, Degens P, Sander I [1998]. Baker's asthma: still amongst the most frequent occupational respiratory disorders. J All Clin Immunol 102(6 Pt 1):984–997.

Biagini RE, MacKenzie BA, Sammons DL, Smith JP, Striley CA, Robertson SK, Snawder JE [2004]. Evaluation of the prevalence of anti-wheat, anti-flour dust, and anti-α-amylase specific IgE antibodies in US blood donors. Ann Allergy Asthma Immun 92(6):649–653.

Bogdanovic J, Wouters IM, Sander I, Zahradnik E, Harris-Roberts J, Rodrigo M, Gomez-Olles S, Heederick DJJ, Goekes G [2006]. Airborne exposure to wheat allergens: optimized elution for airborne dust samples. J Environ Monit 8(10):1043–1048.

Bulat P, Myny K, Braeckman L, van Sprundel M, Kusters E, Doekes G, Pössel K, Droste J, Vanhoorne M [2004]. Exposure to inhalable dust, wheat flour and alpha-amylase allergens in industrial and traditional bakeries. Ann Occup Hyg 48(1):57–63.

CDC [1998]. Guideline for infection control in health care personnel. Am J Infect Control 26(3):289–354.

CFR. Code of Federal Regulations. Washington, DC: U.S. Government Printing Office, Office of the Federal Register.

Cummings KJ, Gaughan DM, Kullman GJ, Beezhold DH, Green BJ, Blachere FM, Bledsoe T, Kreiss K, Cox-Ganser J [2010]. Adverse respiratory outcomes associated with occupational exposures at a soy processing plant. Eur Respir J 36(5):1007–1015.

De Zotti R, Larese F, Bovenzi M, Negro C, Molinari S [1994]. Allergic airway disease in Italian bakers and pastry makers. Occup Environ Med 51(8):548–552.

Elms J, Robinson E, Rahman S, Garrod A [2005]. Exposure to flour dust in UK bakeries: current use of control measures. Ann Occup Hyg *49*(1):85–91.

Gautrin D, Infante-Rivard C, Dao TV, Magnan-Larose M, Desjardins J, Malo JM [1997]. Specific IgE-dependent sensitization, atopy, and bronchial hyperresponsiveness in apprentices starting exposure to protein derived agents. Am J Respir Crit Care Med *155*(6):1841–1847.

Gomez-Olles S, Cruz MJ, Bogdanovic J, Wouters IM, Doekes G, Sander I, Morell F, Rodrigo MJ [2007]. Assessment of soy aeroallergen levels in different work environments. Clin Exp Allergy *37*(12):1863–1872.

Grassi M, Rezzani C, Biino G, Marinoni A [2003]. Asthma-like symptoms assessment through ECRHS screening questionnaire scoring. J Clin Epidem *56*(3):238–247.

Houba R, Heederick D, Doekes G, van Run P [1996]. Exposure sensitization relationship for α-amylase allergens in the baking industry. Am J Respir Crit Care Med *154*(1):130–136.

Houba R, Heederik D, Doekes G [1998a]. Wheat sensitization and work related symptoms in the baking industry are preventable: an epidemiologic study. Am J Respir Crit Care Med *158*(5 Pt 1):1499–1503.

Houba R, Doekes G, Heederick D [1998b]. Occupational respiratory allergy in bakery workers: a review of the literature. Am J Ind Med *34*(6):529–546.

NIOSH [2004]. NIOSH respirator selection logic. Cincinnati, OH: U.S. Department of Health and Human Services, Centers for Disease Control and Prevention, National Institute for Occupational Safety and Health, DHHS (NIOSH) Publication No. 2005-100. [http://www.cdc.gov/niosh/docs/2005-100/pdfs/2005-100.pdf]. Date accessed: April 2013.

NIOSH [2010]. NIOSH pocket guide to chemical hazards. Cincinnati, OH: U.S. Department of Health and Human Services, Centers for Disease Control and Prevention, National Institute for Occupational Safety and Health, DHHS (NIOSH) Publication No. 2010-168c. [http://www.cdc.gov/niosh/npg/]. Date accessed: April 2013.

OSHA [2009]. Assigned protection factors for the revised respiratory protection standard. Washington, D.C. U.S. Department of Labor, Occupational Safety and Health Administration, OSHA 3352-02.

Page EH, Dowell CH, Mueller CA, Biagini RE, Heederick D [2010]. Exposure to flour dust and sensitization among bakery employees. Am J Ind Med *53*(12):1225–32.

Park HS, Nahm DH [1997]. Identification of IgE-binding components in occupational asthma caused by corn dust. Ann Allergy Asthma Immunol *79*(1):75–79.

Sander I, Flagge A, Merget R, Halder TM, Meyer HE, Baur X [2001]. Identification of wheat flour allergens by means of 2-dimensional immunoblotting. J Allergy Clin Immunol *107*(5):907–913.

Schöll I, Jensen-Jarolim E [2004]. Allergenic potency of spices: hot, medium hot, or very hot. Int Arch Allergy Immunol *135*(3):247–261.

Keywords: NAICS 31165 (poultry processing), flour dust, flour, wheat, soy, asthma, sensitization, poultry processing, poultry breading, spices

The Health Hazard Evaluation Program investigates possible health hazards in the workplace under the authority of Section 20(a)(6) of the Occupational Safety and Health Act of 1970, 29 U.S.C. 669(a)(6). The Health Hazard Evaluation Program also provides, upon request, technical assistance to federal, state, and local agencies to control occupational health hazards and to prevent occupational illness and disease. Regulations guiding the Program can be found in Title 42, Code of Federal Regulations, Part 85; Requests for Health Hazard Evaluations (42 CFR 85).

Acknowledgments

Analytical Support: Barbara MacKenzie, DataChem Laboratories, Clayton Group Services, and the Universiteit Utrecht Institute for Risk Assessment Sciences
Desktop Publishers: Greg Hartle and Mary Winfree
Editor: Ellen Galloway
Health Communicator: Stefanie Brown
Industrial Hygiene Field Assistance: Donald Booher, Gregory Burr, Kevin L. Dunn, and Todd Niemeier
Logistics: Karl Feldmann
Medical Field Assistance: Judith Eisenberg, Loren Tapp, Carlos Aristeguieta, Barbara MacKenzie, Deborah Sammons, Gowtham Rao, Shirley Robertson, and John Clark

Availability of Report

Copies of this report have been sent to the employer, employees, and union at the plant. The state and local health department and the Occupational Safety and Health Administration Regional Office have also received a copy. This report is not copyrighted and may be freely reproduced.

This report is available at http://www.cdc.gov/niosh/hhe/reports/pdfs/2009-0131-3171.pdf

Recommended citation for this report:
NIOSH [2013]. Health hazard evaluation report: evaluation of sensitization and exposure to flour dust, spices, and other ingredients among poultry breading workers. By Page EH, Dowell CH, Mueller CA, Biagini RE. Cincinnati, OH: U.S. Department of Health and Human Services, Centers for Disease Control and Prevention, National Institute for Occupational Safety and Health, NIOSH HETA No. 2009-0131-3171.

To receive NIOSH documents or more information about occupational safety and health topics, please contact NIOSH:

Telephone: 1–800–CDC–INFO (1–800–232–4636)

TTY: 1–888–232–6348

CDC INFO: www.cdc.gov/info

or visit the NIOSH Web site at www.cdc.gov/niosh

For a monthly update on news at NIOSH, subscribe to NIOSH eNews by visiting www.cdc.gov/niosh/eNews.

SAFER • HEALTHIER • PEOPLE™

www.ingramcontent.com/pod-product-compliance
Lightning Source LLC
Chambersburg PA
CBHW080924290526
45795CB00007BA/2646